Use Your Mind to Lose Weight

How to use the Law of Attraction to lose weight and get healthy

Jo Story

Use Your Mind to Lose Weight

Table of Contents

Use Your Mind to Lose Weight

Obesity Conversations

"Obesity epidemic"—it's enough to send the feds into a panic and the medical world into research mode to find drugs and other treatments designed to stop this epidemic.

"Ooh, we have to fight against obesity, because it is more dangerous than the worst diseases! Argh!"

And yet...many people are getting bigger, not smaller, and the "fight against obesity" campaign seems to be working in the opposite direction. Television is full of reality shows where obese people fight for their lives by losing weight. The First Lady, Michelle Obama, has made childhood obesity her pet project. So-called "health initiatives" are instituted in schools across the country in the hopes that kids will make "healthier" choices. But instead of having the intended results that they

Use Your Mind to Lose Weight

wanted, the exact opposite is happening. Even when kids make "healthy" choices, they still gain weight and fight off fat constantly. What is going on?

At the government level, nutritional recommendations and policies for food assistance programs are based on the current food guidelines, now in a plate diagram instead of the pyramid diagram. This affects the emergency food pantries, WIC and other food supplemental programs, which forces the poor of the nation to be required to eat food that will make them fight off body fat all their lives. Or does it?

The media talks all the time about the obesity crisis in this nation and other westernized cultures. Diseases stem from obesity; higher healthcare costs exist due to obesity; and the entire culture is changing due to obesity. The talk of obesity never ends, and because everyone is focused on obesity, no one focuses on health. Is it any wonder no one is healthy

Use Your Mind to Lose Weight

when no one focuses on health? It should make perfect sense that since we are focused on obesity, more and more people are getting obese.

People say that eating healthy requires a lot of money. Does it? Really? Fruits, vegetables, dairy and meat are the basics of human health and form the foundation of a healthy existence. If you have a food budget, you have money to buy healthy food. What makes it more expensive is adding processed food and convenience foods to your bill. There is really no need for these extra foods, and if you do not buy them, you can afford the healthy foods. It's all really in how you think about what healthy really is.

Exercise is promoted as a way to lose body fat and get healthy. Even clinical studies are manipulated to somehow "prove" this. Other studies are the opposite; that we don't need to exercise to lose weight, nor do we need to kill ourselves in

Use Your Mind to Lose Weight

the gym just to get healthy. Health clubs love to prey on this misinformation and tell us that we need to join their club just to get healthy and lose weight. They tell us that we are fat and lazy if we don't join their clubs.

Drug companies get in on the action as well. Although, they come at us from the angle that losing weight is very hard and we don't have to struggle alone. That all we need to do is pop a pill every day and not take responsibility for what food we put in our mouths and we will lose weight and be thin. It's interesting to note though that in the small print for the weight loss drug commercials, "Results typical with diet and exercise". Are we stupid? Are we that ridiculously stupid that we will believe that a weight loss drug will make us thin? But they tell us that we are overweight and we need their drugs or we won't reach our goals.

Aside from all this, there are people out there publishing

Use Your Mind to Lose Weight

books (*guilty!*), supplements, and programs all designed for weight loss. They are all telling us that we are fat...that we should lose a few extra pounds...that we will never be good enough or pretty enough or smart enough without their product or program.

Have you had enough yet? Have you had so much of this nonsense that you want to scream? Go ahead and scream then. In fact, I will do it for you! Take a look:

STOP the insane conversations of obesity!!! STOP FEEDING US THIS CRAP! Stop telling us that we are fat, lazy, unhealthy and stupid! Stop telling us that we have to fight obesity! It will never work!!!

Does this make sense to "***fight against***" anything?? What we focus on we bring into our lives. When you focus on how much you want to lose weight, you end up gaining weight. If you lose weight, is it easy, or is it hard? What is your experience?

Use Your Mind to Lose Weight

Chances are that if you are focused on "losing weight" you may inadvertently be causing your weight gain, or at least your struggle with your weight.

The focus here is not that you are fat or lazy, or even stupid. No, this is different than what you may be used to for a "weight loss" book. Instead of talking about what you should or shouldn't do, we are focusing on what you are thinking about yourself, where you got your ideas from and what you are doing with those ideas.

But first, you should know who I am, where I have been, where I am going, and why I am qualified to talk about this topic with authority.

Use Your Mind to Lose Weight

My Story

At the age of 32, I thought I had it together. Husband, kids, nice house, new car—yep, I had the good life. I even went through some transformational work and worked on who I was. During that time, I had also lost quite a bit of weight—56 pounds, to be exact. I even wrote a couple books, explaining how I did it. Boy, I was going somewhere, to be sure! It didn't last long, and soon, I was depressed again and back to the weight I was before losing all that weight. Two and a half years later, my marriage broke up and the kids and I relocated to a small town in Wisconsin. Having had to give up the new car, I had to settle for an old car with plenty of problems. The weight climbed even higher to an astounding 360 pounds!

How in the world did I get here after having it all? Why did my weight go up so high? I was depressed, plain and simple. I

Use Your Mind to Lose Weight

forgot all the lessons I learned about losing weight, and I was stuck in the language that I was fat once again. Well, to be honest, I didn't even care about my weight anymore—it was way down on my list of things to worry about after my life turned upside down. Healing my mind and my children came first. After all, if the mind is not whole, the body will not be whole. This is the first and foremost lesson to learn—keep your mind balanced and your body will follow.

I wrote a book, The Art of Language for Weight Loss around the time that I lost all that weight the first time, detailing the internal thought processes that make losing weight so much simpler. I told the story of how I came to realize that I was using the language of being fat to stay fat and to stop trying to be thin. However, there is more to the story.

Shortly after writing that book and losing the weight, we

Use Your Mind to Lose Weight

moved to Minnesota away from the home that I loved to a home that bled us dry financially and emotionally. I tried keeping up the weight loss, but I found it too difficult to keep at it, especially because I tried cutting out all flesh and flesh-based foods. *Otherwise known as a "vegan" diet.* It was a nightmare to keep going and I had to have meat and dairy again. But I didn't know how to incorporate it back without gaining the weight again, and I slowly gained all the weight I lost.

My marriage was coming to the end, which also contributed to my emotional distress and weight gain. For many years, I had been raped and controlled to the point of humiliation. I was depressed and too upset to continue losing weight. As a way to stop the pain and the humiliation, I tried a unique way of getting out of the marriage—a sex change. Several days before "coming out" as transgender, I remember thinking that if I was

Use Your Mind to Lose Weight

a man, he wouldn't be able to hurt me anymore and I could be strong again. That is what I did. The language that went along with that was that if I were a man, I wouldn't have to worry about my weight and I could eat what I wanted with nothing to stop me. Hmmm...now the language was fully and completely set up to make me fat. I no longer cared about my body and appearance, and I gave in to my cravings. It was a brutal language that matched brutal times.

When my marriage finally ended in 2008, I weighed 275, up from 204 pounds just 2½ years earlier. I gained back 71 pounds! I was appalled at myself, and literally disgusted with how big I got. But I still did not care—who would after all the crap I went through? I had bigger things to worry about and I was not about to start caring about my size just yet. Once relocating to my current small town, I put on an additional 85 pounds in one

Use Your Mind to Lose Weight

year, bringing my weight to an astounding 360 pounds on a 5'8" frame. "Ouch" would be the correct word for this. Eventually, I started caring about my weight, but I didn't know what could work to really start getting my weight down to a manageable level.

I continued researching and learning what really could help me lose weight. It wasn't through a vegan or vegetarian diet; nor was it a low fat, high carbohydrate diet. What I learned was that Dr. Atkins had it right when it came to weight loss—that limiting carbohydrates in favor of saturated fats and proteins was the way to go. Was I ready to start this yet? <u>Uh...no.</u> I **loved** my grains and starchy foods. I didn't want to give up my soda and sweets, and I stayed stuck.

By late 2009, I decided I was ready to start losing weight, and I was going to do it the low-carb way. I started having more meat than anything else...and it worked, up until the holidays. I

Use Your Mind to Lose Weight

lost 20 pounds in a few short weeks, but when Thanksgiving rolled around, I gave up. I wanted to do up the meal just right and not worry about watching my weight. This happened at Christmas as well, making me gain all 20 pounds back.

I researched more into the low carb way of eating and found out many things that I will talk about in other e-books along the way. Apparently, this way of eating was the accepted practice more than 100 years ago to help people lose weight, which makes it not such a "new" fad diet.

Convinced that I could finally lose weight and armed with a great plan in place, I ventured forward. In the middle of May 2010, I started a very low carb lifestyle. Two short weeks later, I had dropped to 345—at a loss of 15 pounds. I was excited—if this is what it does, I definitely want to continue! I began living the language of weight loss possibilities. I continued and by

Use Your Mind to Lose Weight

June 1, 2010, I took grains out of my diet in favor of nuts and seeds. That summer, I lost a total of 65 pounds. By the time fall came, I weighed 280 pounds, just in time to move to a different place in the same small town.

However, with moving and winter/holidays, I ended up putting back on some of the weight. I lost the language for weight loss and the weight came back—but not all of it. In fact, I only gained 25 pounds, making my net loss of 40 pounds. Still, this was disturbing to me, as I wanted to at least maintain the loss. A lot of things happened that winter and I forgot what I had written about weight loss several years back. I got back into the "I'm fat" language, and lo and behold, I began going that direction.

Again, I wanted to get the weight off. A couple neighbors wanted to lose weight too, so I dusted off my ideas and got to work. May 1st, 2011, was the

Use Your Mind to Lose Weight

date we were supposed to get started. I half-heartedly put some effort into losing weight, just to humor them. But my mind was not in it... I did lose 10 pounds in a week and a half, though, because I went back to only meat and vegetables. I believe that this was also a result of mentally getting prepared for weight loss. I was in the language of weight loss, which helped me lose those first ten pounds. Finally, on May 13, 2011, I got serious. I got honest with myself and realized that I weighed 305 pounds! Ouch indeed!

That was a net loss of 50 pounds, which in reality, is still a good loss. By the 13th of May, I decided I would kick ass and really start letting go of this weight. That was the beginning of using language to lose weight for 2011. I knew, beyond a shadow of a doubt, that I would lose the neighbors' goal of 30 pounds for the summer, plus more! At this writing, July 25th, 2011, I have made it to 50 pounds gone, for a grand

Use Your Mind to Lose Weight

weight loss total of 100 pounds! I am at 255 pounds, and very happy that it happened so quickly.

Since this time, I lost the language again, however briefly, and the weight loss stopped altogether. See how this works? When you take your eyes away from the language that allows you to get what you want, you lose the momentum and what you want gradually slips away without so much as a "goodbye". I have picked up my language again and am now moving forward at about a ½ to 1-pound loss per day. My final goal is to lose another 100-120 pounds.

Weight loss is not an action—at least initially. You must set yourself up for weight loss…you must be mentally and emotionally stable and balanced to lose weight. It's difficult to maintain your weight, or even lose weight if your mind is focused on the bad in your life. It's also hard to lose weight if you think you are

Use Your Mind to Lose Weight

fat and you will never be anything else but fat. Who said you must be fat through life?

I challenge you to take responsibility for your choice to tell yourself that you are fat and will remain fat for life. You are the one who said you were fat...you were the one who believed every little comment about your size. No one else made you choose that language. You were the one who chose that language, and guess what? You are the one who can choose a different language!

Use Your Mind to Lose Weight

Language Matters

What you say or what you think matters, especially when it comes to weight loss. In my previous book, I outlined that if you want to be thin, you must think thin. In case you have not read that book, here is an excerpt about this topic:

> "I thought in terms of new possibilities and new realities for myself and what I could do. I didn't limit myself, but did as much as I could do, while still challenging myself. **Since I thought thin, I "knew" I could do whatever I set my mind to do.** I had always heard that said to me as I was growing up, but because of the decisions I made

Use Your Mind to Lose Weight

about myself, I thought in the limitations I placed upon myself. (Namely FAT.) That is what held me back all those years, and I am sure that is what is holding you back too. Are you putting limits on what you can do? Let me ask that in another way: Are you only doing what you "know" you can do and no more?? How do you "know" that is all you can do? Are you dead? You can always do more...

"You are putting limits on yourself and your body. Your body is an amazing structure! You may get frustrated with your

Use Your Mind to Lose Weight

body, because it is not doing what you want it to do. Yet you will avoid exercise, eat refined and processed foods, drink either regular or diet sodas, and have snacks that aren't healthy for you in the first place. Am I right? But yet, you want your body to lose 50 pounds, so you can fit into a skimpy little bikini or be buff at the gym, right?

"Thinking thin is only a portion of the weight loss process. As you think of yourself as strong, powerful, and thin, you must think of it as a fact—as something that is as undisputed as your name. Believe it like

Use Your Mind to Lose Weight

your life depends on it. (Actually, it does depend on it.)

"Because you believe it, then you will automatically begin an exercise routine...you will begin to buy healthier foods...you will give up your sodas. You will begin craving the things that are healthy for you, and you will begin hating that stuff that you are consuming right now. But the very first step is to choose how you are being right now. Are you being thin? Are you being strong? Are you being powerful? Are you being healthy? As you are being those, then there is no

Use Your Mind to Lose Weight

struggle. The only struggle you have is the one you choose to make. You make the struggle in your own mind. When you choose to not make losing weight a struggle, there is no suffering and no feeling "bad" about slipping once in a while."

Thinking that you are fat will keep you fat, no matter what you try to do. "Losing weight" thoughts will bring more weight into your life. Obsessing about numbers on a scale or on a measuring tape with drive you nuts with worry and it will keep you from really being free. Trust me, I do this and it is driving me nuts! Every time I step on the scale or use the measuring tape, I try to fudge it a little so the numbers are smaller. This is not entirely helpful in the long term because it is not making me free. It is not giving

Use Your Mind to Lose Weight

me the language I need to truly be free to be healthy and happy.

Let me tell you a tale of two scales. (Trust me, this is related to this topic.) For a long time, I thought that I weighed much less than I really did. That was on my old scale. Then, when I went to my parents' house for a week visit, I stepped on their digital scale and it said that I weighed at least 60 pounds more than I thought I did! Well, of course I never believed it because it did not match up to my old scale back at home. It did, however, plant seeds of doubt in my mind, wondering where I really was in my weight loss journey. I wanted to just stop weight loss altogether because I was too discouraged. Language—it got me again!

For at least a month after getting back home from visiting my parents, I refused to do anything to lose weight or get my health back in line with what I wanted. Because of this, I put on some weight again. The

Use Your Mind to Lose Weight

moment I took my eyes off the prize, so to speak, I lost momentum and took a few steps back. But the scale still said I weighed about 60 pounds less. How did I find this out? Recently, I bought a new scale that is more accurate, because I wanted to find out where I was at so I can go forward again. Getting honest with where you are at can make a big difference in whether you succeed and move forward, or if you stay stuck.

So I bought that new scale, brought it home, took it out of the packaging and set it up in my bathroom. I stepped on it, expecting it to be just a touch above where I thought I was. Nope! It went all the way to where my parents' scale said I was! I was devastated! If that was where I am, then where did I start from at the very beginning? I went into a crisis at this time. I figured out that if I thought I started at 290 pounds in May of 2010, then I must have actually been at 360

Use Your Mind to Lose Weight

pounds! (I figure my old scale was about 60-70 pounds off.)

The other thing that made sense to me was that if I lost about 105 pounds, then this figure was about right. How in the world did I get up that high? This taught me a lesson about obsessing about numbers on the scale or from the measuring tape. When you obsess about numbers, you get caught up in the numbers, taking your eyes off the prize when the numbers are not moving in the direction you want them to. If you feel healthy and you are focusing on living a healthy life, it will all fall into place.

Language really does matter in everything in life. How we think about things, what language we choose, and the tone we choose to live life in determines what comes into our lives. More often than not, we think about what we don't want, and then we bring that into our lives. You may not be thinking you are fat, but you are probably

Use Your Mind to Lose Weight

thinking about how much you don't want to be fat. Guess what? You are bringing that into your life.

It does not matter if you do NOT want what you are thinking about. Only what you don't want to begin with will be listened to and you will have more of the same of what you don't want. If you don't want to be fat, more of being fat will come into your life. Thinking that you want to be healthy and thin will bring more of that into your life. What you think about you manifest in every part of your life. Thinking about how much you don't want something will bring that very thing into your life, because of how much you are thinking about it.

Here's an example: for years, I believed that I was not worth having a romance movie quality relationship. That what I wanted didn't matter because I wasn't going to get it anyway. The relationship I fell into, while it produced three

Use Your Mind to Lose Weight

beautiful children who I absolutely adore and love, became more of a horror movie than a romance movie. Because I did not believe I was worth having a wonderful relationship, I did not have a wonderful relationship. That marriage is done, but I now realize that I deserve a spectacular, loving relationship with the person of my dreams.

Language, the words we use to put ourselves or others down; the words we use to describe the world around us; and the words that we use to describe what we think is true are all working together to create what we get in life. Words create our reality—what we think, what we want, what we don't want— every single part of our reality is shaped by the language we use. Now you can say, "I don't believe that. That sounds like new-age hogwash." Let me ask you something. What happened the last time you made a major change in your life for the betterment of your life? Did it just happen? Did someone else

Use Your Mind to Lose Weight

create that change for you? Or, did you begin to think about wanting something and then figured out a way for it to happen?

Chances are, you thought about it first. You began studying and researching into how to make it happen. Then you started taking actions to make it happen—slowly at first—but then it gained momentum.

That, my dear friend, is what I am talking about here. Thoughts shape who we are and what we are about. When you think in a negative way, your entire life becomes negative. This is more than just having a positive outlook. Some people, when accused of being negative, say, "I am just mirroring what society gave me." Or, is it the other way around—that you became a mirror to society and it gave you what you thought about? I do not mean here that you thought about wanting the horrors that you may have endured. I am not blaming you for anything bad that happened in your life. No, this is about how we feel and what we think about ourselves and about the world around us.

Let's put this into perspective for a moment. Say, as a child, you grew up in poverty and there was nothing you could do about it. Everyone around you that you trusted made sure you knew that poverty happens because the rich people are selfish and do not want to share the wealth. Or that it is impossible to get ahead in this world and you might as well give up trying. If that is what you were told as a child, you will believe this to be true because you are looking for it to be true. The language that you use here will shape your future because you just KNOW it is true. What if it isn't true though? What if, instead of focusing on how poor you are, you start focusing on gratitude for what you have? Focus for just a moment on how lucky you are to be alive? Carry that

Use Your Mind to Lose Weight

one thought with you and see what happens. More good feelings and experiences will come to you because you are now focusing on the good feelings of appreciation.

What does this have to do with losing weight? Whatever you want it to mean, right? Well, let me tell you what it has to do with weight loss from my own perspective.

As I have mentioned earlier, my language created the mess I was in. When I lived in the language of being healthy, my actions aligned with being healthy. When I lived in the language of "I don't care. It's not working anyway", then my actions aligned with not caring and I got the results of not caring—gaining weight and being unhealthy. Being healthy requires that you let your thoughts be healthy and aligned with what is possible. Staying stuck in the language that got you fat in the first place will keep you fat and, potentially, unhealthy. This is

Use Your Mind to Lose Weight

not a place I want to be in, and I don't think you want to be in this place either. Get out of the language that keeps you stuck and in the language that allows you to move forward.

Use Your Mind to Lose Weight

No More Labels

Labels belong on things, not people. Therefore, take every single label you have put on yourself or that others have put on you and throw them away. Get rid of them right now! What labels am I talking about? When someone tells you that you are a certain way, such as hard working, stubborn, bright, selfish, loving, greedy, smart, independent, or even attractive, these are labels. They are putting you into a box that has you acting or behaving in a certain way. This is not who you are, nor who you have to be. These labels are what make you do certain things and have certain things in your life. They are not entirely helpful, are they?

I dare say that labels are what made you gain weight, right? Perhaps in life you were told that you were fat or that you were just destined to fight your weight because that was what other people in your family have done. It becomes the "truth". But it is not the truth— it is only one way of seeing things. Weight issues run in families, not because of genes or being "pre-destined" to be fat, but because the labels or language that live in families says that they are supposed to have weight problems. It's an almost pre-programmed way of life and, to escape the language, you have to throw away the destructive language.

Truth is a subjective idea. The more evidence you have about a certain idea, the more it becomes real. Likewise, the more agreement you have with other people, the more it must be true. So you're fat because there is agreement and evidence that you have to be this way? I don't think so! You don't have to stay this way, do you?

"I can't lose weight." Can't? Or won't? The question is not whether you have the ability to lose weight or not, but whether you will take the actions

Use Your Mind to Lose Weight

necessary to achieve your goals. Throwing off the label that you are fat forces you to rethink your ideas or reasons why you have to stay stuck. Labels got you where you are, correct? Labels like "fat", "unhealthy", "unmotivated", or even "poor" can throw off your thoughts and keep you where you are. You are not your labels. Throw away your labels and get rid of negative thoughts and actions.

Labels got you unhealthy. Poor you. You are so unhealthy. You can't do anything about your situation, because this is how it has always been. You can't be healthy because you are poor and cannot afford quality food. These labels are harmful and will keep you stuck in an unhealthy way of life that will not allow you to go forward and get to your goals of healthy and thin.

Labels make you stay stuck and not even try. Either that, or they make you try too hard, giving you disastrous results. If you try too hard and you fail,

Use Your Mind to Lose Weight

you will be that much more likely to go to either extreme. Either you will increase your efforts so much that you become anorexic, or you will stop all efforts and become morbidly obese. Labels will not allow you to get past unhealthy habits.

Throw away all labels and start fresh. Believe that you are worth the effort you put forth to get healthy and happy. Begin feeling right now the magic of success and healthy habits. Imagine yourself going through the steps it will take to be healthy. Enjoy the feelings of health, vitality and energy. Live life like it is true for you right now. Only then will you find the success you crave so much!

Again—THROW AWAY THE LABELS!!!

Use Your Mind to Lose Weight

Take Responsibility for your Thoughts

Only you can tell yourself what to think. No one else has that power over you, no matter what other people want to think. When I was married, my spouse would tell me what he wanted me to think, how to act and who to be. Think that was bad? No, the worse part was that I actually let him do that to me! While he could not control my inner thoughts, the words he used and the language of life he lived in created that control over me. Everything that I thought about myself and my life was a direct result of what he would say and think about me. I lost every part of me that I loved. I lost my inner soul because of the language that he used about me. I did not take responsibility for my thoughts. I was at the whim of someone else's thoughts and I did not realize it.

Use Your Mind to Lose Weight

When you have conversations coming at you from all sides about obesity, it's pretty hard to not think about obesity, losing weight and getting thin. But that only perpetuates obesity and disease. That creates thoughts within you that you cannot lose weight easily and that you are lazy if you do not work to change your body. When the conversation at the government level talks about how fat we all are...when the conversation on TV says we are fat...when health clubs want us to sign up for membership so they can make money...all these are pretty big influences on what you think about yourself and how fat you are.

This is utter nonsense. You do not have to give in to these conversations. You have a brain. You have intelligence. You do not need to think the way everyone else wants you to think. When you give in to these conversations, you are saying about yourself, "I do not matter. I am not smart enough to figure my way out of my

Use Your Mind to Lose Weight

situation. Other people are smarter than me and they need to help me get out of this mess I created for myself." Do you really want to think that about yourself? Then stop listening to those conversations!

No one else lives in your head. They aren't telling you what to think, so take responsibility for your thoughts. You are the one that has control over what comes into your mind. There are 86,400 seconds in a day, which means there are 86,400 chances per day to think of what you want to have happen in your life. Of course, there are also 86,400 chances to still screw up your life with your thoughts too. Your choice, isn't it?

You must get now that you are the only person who can think your thoughts; feel your feelings; choose your choices. You can choose to believe the obesity conversations, or you can choose to believe your own conversations about what you want for you. Your life does not

Use Your Mind to Lose Weight

have to go the way of someone else's choosing for you. Instead, you can choose an entirely different path and think for yourself. Take responsibility for your thoughts, because if you don't, who will?

Use Your Mind to Lose Weight

Thoughts...Feelings... Actions!

Have you ever had a thought and then felt just awful about it? Or maybe you had a thought and you felt giddy and on top of the world. What did you do after those thoughts and the resulting feelings? Chances are you acted upon how you felt. If you were sad, you probably curled up on the couch, put on a sad movie on TV and ate some comfort food. Maybe if you were happy, you would go out and do something fun, without the comfort food. Then again, you most likely celebrated good news with food. I don't know—I am making this up as I go along. But this is what most people do, and it's what I did for several years. What you thought influenced your feelings, which in turn influences your actions. Those actions influence more thoughts, feelings and actions until your life is either the way you want it to be or it is a mess,

Use Your Mind to Lose Weight

or anything in between these two extremes.

Do thoughts influence feelings? Do feelings influence thoughts? Do actions influence thoughts and feelings? Actually, they all work together in tandem, with one leading to the next. It's really like a spider web in that it's all connected. What we feel leads to what we think, and what we think leads to what we do. But you say, "Feelings are not controllable!" Really? Have you ever had enough of your bad feelings and decided to feel good? **In that moment** you decide to feel good, what happens? You begin to feel your mood lifting and it's like the clouds roll away, letting the sunshine in. Yes, you control your feelings—your feelings do not control you. If this sounds radical and "out there", then you are most likely not used to being in control of your emotions.

Transfer this concept to the practical now...look back at the years where you put on weight.

Use Your Mind to Lose Weight

All the times that you ate when you weren't really hungry, or you mindlessly watched TV while putting snacks into your mouth—what were you feeling? What were you thinking? Feelings of boredom, sadness, anger, happiness, peace, contentment, hopelessness, and many others lead to corresponding thoughts. Feelings of anger lead to angry thoughts, while feelings of sadness lead to sad thoughts. These thoughts lead to actions that match, creating the life you have. If you were sad and your thought to accompany that feeling was that you deserved the bowl of ice cream, then you will go get that bowl of ice cream. Eating ice cream is not a crime, nor will one bowl of the stuff make you gain a lot of weight. Recognizing that what you felt led to a thought that gave way to action is more than half the battle—it is the battle.

Feelings and thoughts are intertwined with actions. If you feel that you are worthless and thoughts confirm this feeling,

Use Your Mind to Lose Weight

then you will act like you are worthless. Likewise, when you feel that you are valuable and think thoughts that confirm this feeling, you will act like you are valuable. You will treat yourself differently. You will give yourself several opportunities to show that you are valuable in how you take care of yourself and how you treat others in your life.

Getting fit and healthy are actions that show this—that you are valuable and worth caring for. This may be why you have struggled with getting rid of excess body weight and why you wanted to blame everything and everyone else for your thoughts about yourself. As was pointed out before, you and only you are responsible for your thoughts. No one else can think your thoughts and feel your feelings.

Now, try this—force yourself to feel valuable. Feel what it would be like to have people hanging on your every word and getting a blessing from what you say.

Use Your Mind to Lose Weight

Think about the many lessons you have learned in life and how you could share that with the world. What are the actions you would take because of this feeling and this thought?

Or, force yourself to feel happy. Feelings of happiness and joy lead to happy thoughts, happy actions and a life you love. Just feeling happy can give you power and energy. Naturally, you will want to be active and do things that will enrich your life. You will begin to care about yourself and do what it takes to be happy.

I hope you have learned a lot from this short time you took with me to read this book. Only YOU have the power to choose what to think, how to act and what to feel. Applying this to your health can make the difference between staying where you are at and moving into alignment with where you want to be. Align your thoughts with what you want and you will have it. Sounds too simple? It is, but it works. Give it a try

Use Your Mind to Lose Weight

and I will see you on the other side!